WHAT IS NEUROPATHIC PAIN?

Neuropathic pain is caused by damage or injury to the nerves that move data between the brain and spinal cord from the skin, muscles and other parts of the body.

The pain is usually depicted as a burning sensation and affected regions are frequently delicate to the contact. Symptoms of neuropathic torment may additionally include excruciating torment, pins and needles, difficulty correctly sensing temperatures and numbness.

Some people may find it hard to wear thick clothes as even slight pressure can exasperate the pain.

Neuropathic Pain is a complex, chronic torment state that typically is accompanied by tissue injury. With neuropathic pain, the nerve fibers themselves might be damaged, dysfunctional, or injured. These harmed nerve filaments send wrong motions toward other pain focuses. The impact of a nerve fiber injury includes a change in nerve function both at the site of injury and areas around the injury.

Neuropathic torment - in any case known as nerve torment - is a type of chronic pain that occurs when nerves in the focal nervous system become injured or damaged.

If you or someone you care about has nerve pain, you know that it can erode quality of life.

TYPES OF NEUROPATHIC PAIN

Entrapment Neuropathy

A caught or pinched nerve at the neck, shoulder, elbow, wrist, hip, lower leg, or foot. Common examples of nerve ensnarement include carpal tunnel condition, thoracic outlet disorder (neck), or piriformis disorder (hip).

Peripheral Neuropathy

Peripheral neuropathy first develops in the longest nerves of the body in a "glove and stocking" distribution to the hands and feet.

There are various causes of peripheral neuropathy, including certain hereditary conditions, viral diseases, liver or kidney failure, and toxins, as well as diseases such as diabetes, vascular disease, and rheumatoid conditions.

Peripheral neuropathy can be motor, sensory or autonomic in nature.

Phantom Limb Pain

Phantom limb torment occurs in certain individuals after the amputation of an arm or leg. Although the exact cause of phantom limb torment is unknown, it appears to result when the nerves and the brain send faulty signals to the appendage as the hardware attempts to "rewire" itself.

Post Herpetic Neuralgia (PHN)

Post-herpetic neuralgia (PHN) is a type of nerve torment that can occur following a viral infection of herpes zoster "shingles" in the nervous system.

Post herpetic neuralgia aching or cutting pain occurs in regions where the shingles rash developed. The skin in such areas may feel extra sensitive, especially in white-colored scars.

Post Traumatic Neuropathy

Post Traumatic Neuropathy happens after injury or medical strategies, such as surgery or infusion. Nerve torment side effects may arise at the injury site and nerve path.

Trigeminal Neurlagia

Trigeminal neuralgia (TN) is a cause of extreme pain in the face and jaw. Shocking, electric "lightning" pains typically precede dull throbbing agony. Trigeminal neuralgia usually affects only one side of the face.

The exact cause of trigeminal neuralgia is unknown, however it develops where the trigeminal nerve is compacted, pinched, or irritated.

CLINICAL FEATURES OF NEUROPATHIC PAIN

Patients frequently find it difficult to describe the nature of NP; it is outside their previous experience of torment. Sensory loss may be mild and overshadowed by allodynia (all upgrades creating pain), hyperalgesia and hyperpathia (postponed perception, summation and painful aftersensation).

'Rarely, (e.g. trigeminal neuralgia) there is no evident sensory loss. There may be signs of sympathetic brokenness, and occasionally dystrophic changes.

The onset of pain may be delayed, the commonest example being focal poststroke pain (thalamic), which may start months or years after the initiating stroke.

Pain is often of mixed nociceptive and neuropathic types, for model, mechanical spinal pain with radiculopathy or myelopathy. It isn't for the most part perceived that nociceptive spinal pain can radiate generally, copying a root distribution. It can be troublesome to identify the prevailing pain type and treat appropriately. Such patients require careful examination, imaging and neurophysiological investigation.

PATHOPHYSIOLOGY OF NEUROPATHIC PAIN

The pathophysiological properties that are answerable for NP can be comprehensively arranged into five gatherings: ectopic motivation generation in damaged primary afferent fibres, fibre interactions, central sensitisation, disinhibition (disappointment or decrease of normal inhibitory mechanisms), and versatility (degenerative and regenerative changes related with adjusted connectivity).

The mechanisms of NP are considerably unique to those of nociceptive pain.

Novel impulse generators develop at various sites, and these are not upgrade dependent.

In peripheral nerve, it has been shown that ectopic drive generation (EIG) creates as an outcome of the articulation of unusual sodium channels. This can be altered by neurotrophic growth factors (a potential target for new treatments).

Abnormal chemical awarenesses develop in damaged primary sensory neurons, prominently to catecholamines. Whilst this can be readily showed in exploratory preparations, the clinical relevance remains uncertain.

Degenerative and then regenerative changes in the spinal line may lead to unusual connectivity, and potentially a forever reorganised, irreversible state.

Damage at one level in the anxious system may lead to optional pathophysiological changes at more rostral levels. This has important implications when targeting treatments for NP.

ASSESSMENT OF NEUROPATHIC PAIN

Screening questionnaires are suitable for distinguishing potential patients with neuropathic pain, however further validation of them is needed for epidemiological purposes.

Clinical assessment, including precise sensory assessment, is the basis of neuropathic pain diagnosis. For more accurate sensory profiling, quantitative sensory testing is recommended for chosen cases in clinic, including the diagnosis of small fiber neuropathies and for research purposes.

Step 1.

A clinical history of sickness or lesion of the somatosensory framework proposes a possible diagnosis of neuropathic pain

Step 2.

Confirmation by either clinically reproducible signs or investigations would suggest a probable diagnosis of neuropathic pain

Step 3.

If the history, clinical examination and investigations are positive, this would support an unequivocal finding of neuropathic pain

Sensory assessment - light touch, temperature, painful stimulus, vibration and proprioception. Engine testing tone, strength, reflexes and coordination. Look for autonomic changes in colour, temperature, perspiring and swelling.

Examination of a Patient with Peripheral Neuropathic Pain shows a real patient with multiple mononeuropathy due to isolated peripheral nervous framework vasculitis. He is experiencing neuropathic pain in his left hand and both legs.

Functional assessment and sensory and motor examination of both upper and lower limbs is demonstrated. DN4 questionnaire helps with neuropathic pain assessment

Use when neuropathic pain is suspected

MANAGEMENT OF NEUROPATHIC PAIN

Unfortunately, neuropathic torment often responds ineffectively to standard pain treatments and every so often may deteriorate instead of better over time. For some people, it can lead to serious disability.

A multidisciplinary approach that joins treatments, however, can be an exceptionally successful way to provide relief from neuropathic pain.

Other kinds of medicines can also help with neuropathic pain. Some of these include:

- Physical therapy
- Counselling
- Relaxation
- therapy Massage
- therapy Acupuncture

MEDICAL MANAGEMENT

Anticonvulsant and antidepressant drugs for instance, pregabalin, gabapentin and amitriptyline may work to reduce symptoms in most cases. Some neuropathic pain studies suggest the use of non-steroidal anti-inflammatory drugs, such as Aleve or Motrin, may ease pain.

Additionally, some people may require a stronger painkiller, such as those containing morphine and can be utilized if the patient does not answer other therapies.

If another condition, such as diabetes, is involved, better management of that disorder may alleviate the pain. Powerful administration of the condition can likewise help prevent further nerve damage. In cases that are troublesome to treat, a pain expert may use a invasive or implantable gadget to effectively manage the pain.

Electrical stimulation of the nerves involved in neuropathic pain may significantly control the pain symptoms.

PHYSICAL THERAPY MANAGEMENT

TENS is compelling in the treatment of agonizing peripheral neuropathy, and very low level laser therapy has been displayed to be effective in patients with neuropathic pain.

Neurostimulation methods including transcranial attractive excitement (TMS) and cortical electrical stimulation (CES), spinal cord stimulation (SCS) and deep brain stimulation (DBS) have also been found viable in the treatment of neuropathic pain.

In general, profound warming agents like ultrasound and short wave diathermy are not recommended in the treatment of neuropathic pain.

Exercising for just 30 minutes a day on at least three or four days a week will help you with chronic pain management by increasing:

- Muscle
- Strength
- Endurance
- Stability in the joints
- Flexibility in the muscles and joints

Keeping a consistent exercise routine will additionally help control torment. Regular therapeutic exercise will help you keep up with the capacity to move and work actually, instead of becoming disabled by your chronic pain.

There are studies showing that practice may be an significant part of the treatment and prevention of neuropathic pain after chemotherapy. Albeit more information is required and detailed practice remedies do not yet exist for patients receiving cancer treatment.

It has been also found that physical exercise, such as forced treadmill running and swimming, can sufficiently work on mechanical allodynia and heat hyperalgesia in animal models of neuropathic pain.

Although there is not much research on this subject, some article focuses out that low level laser therapy could help in the treatment of neuropathic pain.

Physical therapy tackles the physical side of the inflammation, stiffness, and soreness with exercise, manipulation, and massage, however it also works to help the body recuperate itself by encouraging the development of the body's natural pain-relieving chemicals. This two-pronged approach is what helps make physical therapy so compelling as a pain treatment

MORE ABOUT THE NATURE OF NEUROPATHIC PAIN

Related to the pain there may also be:

Allodynia: This implies that the torment comes on, or becomes worse, with a touch or stimulus that would not normally cause torment. For example, a slight touch on the face may trigger pain if you have trigeminal neuralgia, or the pressure of the bedclothes may set off pain if you have diabetic neuropathy.

Hyperalgesia: This implies that you get severe pain from a boost or contact that would ordinarily cause just slight discomfort. For example, a gentle prod on the painful region might cause extreme pain.

Paraesthesia: This means that you get unpleasant or painful feelings even when there is nothing contacting you, and no stimulus. For instance, you may have painful pins and needles, or electric shock-like sensations.

In addition to the pain itself, the impact that the pain has on your life may be similarly as important. For model, the torment may lead to upset sleep, anxiety and depression.

HOW COMMON IS NEUROPATHIC PAIN?

It is estimated that about 7 in every 100 people in the UK have persistent (chronic) neuropathic torment. It is much more normal in older people who are more likely to develop the conditions listed above.

WHAT IS THE TREATMENT FOR NEUROPATHIC PAIN?

Many patients try traditional pain medication and calming medications that are available over-the-counter. However, these prescriptions are often ineffective for neuropathic pain. On the off chance that the cause of a patient's torment can be distinguished and reversed, correction or the executives of the problem may lead to nerve recovery and diminished torment. However, it might take a extended period of time (months to years) for this process to happen.

When a patients' condition cannot be reversed or effectively made due, pain control using an assortment of medications may be warranted.

Tricyclic antidepressants, including amitriptyline, nortriptyline, desipramine, and imipramine, have shown positive results for the treatment of pain related to diabetic neuropathy, herpes zoster contamination, agonizing polyneuropathy, and postmasectomy pain.

However, these meds have not been displayed to relieve neuropathic torment related with phantom appendage pain, torment related to cancer, chronic lumbar root neuropathic torment, pain related to chemotherapy treatment, or pain related to HIV infection.

Serotonin-norepinephrine reuptake inhibitors including duloxetine and venlafaxine have been examined for the treatment of neuropathic pain. These prescriptions are considered first-line treatment options for torment related to diabetic neuropathy. Venlafaxine has also been shown to be effective for pain management of excruciating polyneuropathies.

Calcium channel alpha-2-delta ligands, including gabapentin and pregabalin, might be effective for pain resulting from diabetic neuropathy and post-herpetic neuropathy.

Topical agents, including topical lidocane and capsaicin, may be recommended to patients with limited peripheral neuropathic pain. These topical specialists are available in gel or patch form.

Opioids (narcotics), such as codeine and morphine, are generally not utilized as first-line treatment for neuropathic torment as there are a number of genuine side impacts to their use, including enslavement and impaired mental functioning, among others.

However, studies have shown that they are effective for the treatment of diabetic fringe neuropathy, post-herpetic neuropathy, painful polyneuropathy, and phantom limb pain.

Another drug, tramadol, is similar to narcotics and has shown positive results for the treatment of diabetic neuropathy, post-herpetic neuropathy, painful polyneuropathy, and apparition limb torment. Tramadol is associated with a lower chance of dependence than typical opioids and is additionally less sedating.

The use of Botox (botulinum toxin type A) has shown positive results for the treatment of pain related to diabetic neuropathy. However, additional research, on a larger scale, is justified to determine its role in the treatment of this type of pain.

Treatments include:

- Medicines.
- Physical treatments.
- Psychological treatments.
- Treating the underlying cause

If this is conceivable, it might help to ease the torment. For example, if you have diabetic neuropathy then good control of the diabetes may help to ease the condition. On the off chance that you have disease, if this can be treated then this may ease the pain.

Note: the seriousness of the torment frequently does not correspond with the seriousness of the underlying condition. For example, pain following shingles (postherpetic neuralgia) can cause a serious pain, even though there is no rash or sign of infection remaining.

MEDICINES USED TO

TREAT NEUROPATHIC PAIN

Commonly used traditional painkillers

You may have as of now tried traditional painkillers such as paracetamol or mitigating painkillers such as ibuprofen that you can purchase from pharmacies. However, these are far-fetched to ease neuropathic torment especially in most cases.

Tricyclic antidepressant medicines

A antidepressant medication in the tricyclic group is a typical treatment for neuropathic pain. It is not used here to treat depression. Tricyclic antidepressants ease neuropathic pain separate to their activity on depression.

It is thought that they work by interfering with the way nerve impulses are transmitted. There are several tricyclic antidepressants yet amitriptyline is the one most commonly used for neuralgic pain.

A tricyclic energizer may ease the pain within a few days however it may take 2-3 weeks. It can take several weeks before you have maximum benefit. Some people give up on their treatment too early. It is best to persevere for at least 4-6 weeks to see how well the antidepressant is working.

Tricyclic antidepressants sometimes cause sluggishness as a side-effect. This often eases in time. To try to keep away from drowsiness, a low portion is usually begun at first and is then built up steadily if needed. Also, the full daily dose is often taken at night because of the drowsiness side-effect.

A dry mouth is another normal side-effect. Frequent tastes of water may help with a dry mouth. See the leaflet that comes with the medicine packet for a full rundown of conceivable side-effects.

Other antidepressant medicines

An energizer called duloxetine has also been shown in research preliminaries to be good at facilitating neuropathic pain. Specifically, duloxetine has been found to be a good treatment for diabetic neuropathy and is now frequently used first-line for this condition.

Duloxetine is not classed as a tricyclic antidepressant yet as a serotonin and norepinephrine reuptake inhibitor (SNRI). It may be tried for different sorts of neuropathic pain if a tricyclic antidepressant has not functioned admirably, or has caused problematic secondary effects. The range of conceivable secondary effects caused by duloxetine is different to those caused by tricyclic antidepressants.

Anti-epileptic medicines (anticonvulsants)

An enemy of epileptic medication, such as gabapentin or pregabalin, is an alternative to an energizer. These medicines are commonly used to treat epilepsy yet they have also been found to ease nerve pain.

An enemy of epileptic medication can stop nerve impulses causing pains separate to its action on preventing epileptic fits (seizures). As with antidepressants, a low portion is usually began at first and built up continuously, if necessary. It might take several weeks for maximum effect as the dose is gradually increased.

Opiate painkillers

Opiate painkillers, such as codeine, morphine and related medicines, are the stronger conventional pain relievers. As a general rule, they are not utilized first-line for neuropathic pain. This is partly because there is a risk of problems of medication reliance, impeded mental functioning and opposite aftereffects with the
long haul use of opiates.

Tramadol is a painkiller that is similar to sedatives yet has an unmistakable method of
action that is different to other narcotic painkillers. Tramadol can be utilized for short-term treatment of neuropathic torment. Tramadol should not be utilized for delayed treatment.

COMBINATIONS OF MEDICINES

Sometimes both a stimulant and an anti-epileptic medication are taken if either alone does not work very well. Sometimes tramadol is consolidated with an energizer or a anti-epileptic medicine.

As they work in different ways, they may complement each other and have a additive effect on easing pain better than either alone.

Capsaicin cream

This is sometimes used to ease pain if the above medicines do not help, or cannot be used in light of the fact that of problems or side-effects. Capsaicin is thought to work by blocking nerves from sending pain messages. Capsaicin cream is applied 3-4 times a day. It can take up to 10 days for a good torment alleviating impact to occur.

Capsaicin can cause an intense consuming feeling when it is applied. Specifically, if it is used less than 3-4 times a day, or if it is applied soon after taking a hot bath or shower.

However, this side-effect tends to dial down with regular use. Capsaicin cream ought to not be applied to broken or inflamed skin. Wash your hands promptly after applying capsaicin cream.

Other medicines

Some other medicines are sometimes used on the counsel of an expert in an aggravation facility. These (for example, ketamine injections) may be an choice if the
above drugs do not help. Ketamine is typically used as a anaesthetic however at low doses it can have a pain-relieving effect.

Another example is lidocaine gel. This is applied to skin, with a unique fix. It is sometimes used for pain following shingles (postherpetic neuralgia). However, note, it needs to be put on to non-disturbed or healed skin.

SIDE-EFFECTS AND TITRATING THE DOSAGE OF MEDICINES

For most of the medicines recorded above it is common practice to start at a low dose at first. This may be adequate to ease the torment however often the portion needs to be expanded if the effect is not good. This is usually done gradually and is called titrating the dose.

Any increase in portion may be started after a certain number of days or weeks - depending on the medicine. Your specialist will advise as to how and when to increase the portion if required; also, the most extreme portion that can be taken for each particular medicine.

The aim is to find the lowest dose required to ease the pain. This is because the lower the portion, the less likely that aftereffects will be troublesome. Possible incidental effects vary for the different drugs used.

A full list of conceivable side-effects can be found with information in the medicine packet. Some people don't develop any aftereffects; certain individuals are only mildly troubled by side-effects that are OK to live with.

However, some people are troubled quite badly by side-effects. Tell your doctor if you develop any irksome side-effects. A change to a different medicine may be an option if this occurs.

PHYSICAL TREATMENTS

Depending on the site and cause of the torment, a specialist in an aggravation facility may exhort one or more actual medicines. These include: physiotherapy, needle therapy, nerve blocks with infused neighborhood anaesthetics, percutaneous electrical nerve stimulation (PENS) and transcutaneous electrical nerve excitement (TENS) machines.

PSYCHOLOGICAL TREATMENTS

Pain can be made more awful by stress, uneasiness and depression. Also, the feeling (perception) of torment can vary relying upon how we react to our torment and conditions. Where pertinent, therapy for anxiety or discouragement may help.

Also, treatments, for example, stress management, counselling, cognitive behavioural therapy, and pain the board programmes sometimes play a part in helping people with persistent (persistent) neuropathic pain.

WHAT IS CBD

If you don't live under a rock, then you know what Cannabis is: the most widely used "recreational drug" in the world, besides alcohol. It has been a subject of focus in light pop culture, dark drug wars, and every area in between.

We all know that it's in fact illegal and that it can get you high, and the assumption is prevalent that the latter has resulted in the former, however this is not so.

Cannabis is not illegal because it can get you high, yet because in the 1930s, big industry lobbied the government to outlaw hemp in any form because it directly threatened their long-established business models with its extremely-efficient applications in paper, textiles, biodegradable plastics, paint, biofuel, horticulture and animal feed, building materials including insulation, and medication among others.

So what is Cannabis, and why is it so useful

WHAT IS CANNABIS

Cannabis is a genus of flowering plant that has three subspecies: Cannabis Indica, Cannabis Sativa, and Cannabis Ruderalis.

The first two species are generally referred to as Marijuana, and have been bred over time to have higher concentrations of THC, which is the cannabinoid that produces the "high" when consumed.

The third species, Cannabis Ruderalis, is a small wild weed that has low levels of any cannabinoids.

Hemp refers to member of a subspecies of sativa that have less than 0.3% THC. That is the defining characteristic, yet it can have a high concentration of CBD which really inhibits the effect of THC on receptors in the brain.

The word Hemp is only used for Cannabis plants and products that have no meaningful amount of THC, and some state run administrations even direct the use of this word.

Hemp is notable primarily because it comprise of a fibrous material that is stronger and cheaper to produce than cotton, has more prominent insulatory properties than fiberglass, more tensile strength than steel cables, and can grow in nearly any non-arctic environment.

WHAT ARE

CANNABINOIDS

Cannabinoids are chemicals found within the Cannabis plant that have some sort of effect on the endocannabinoid system found in all mammals.

Endocannabinoid simply means "cannabinoid inside"; that's right, your body and every mammalian body produces cannabinoids and has an inborn system that responds to them.

Found primarily in the central nervous system, digestive system, and invulnerable framework, we are discovering more and more about the cannabinoid system in your body every day.

What we know so far is that there are over 113 different cannabinoids, two different kinds of receptors, and an limitless number of functions that they serve.

Tetrahydrocannabinol, THC for short, has a number of effects on the body in expansion to producing a high, including strong anti-inflammatory properties.

DEFINING CBD

Cannabidiol, CBD for short, is a wonder of nature to say the least. It is not psychoactive in the basic sense, which means CBD doesn't make you high. It's also a different compound than THC, so it won't show up on a medication test either.

CBD is extracted from the leaves and flowers of cannabis plants, and once it's isolated from the rest of the plant, it can be integrated into a plenty of other products, from sublingual oils, to gummy bears and even topical anti-inflammatory lotion.

By regulating the creations of signals in your cells, acting as an antioxidant, and activating several different types of receptors in your body, CBD is able to exert a number of restorative effects with NO negative side-effects yet discovered.

Combine all of these factors, and it becomes clear that CBD is ultimately an immunostimulant, and has been found to have significant capacity for treating the following symptoms and diseases:

- acne
- ALS
- Alzheimer's disease
- anxiety
- arthritis, including rheumatism
- cancer
- Crohn's disease
- diabetes
- fibromyalgia
- glaucoma
- hepatitis C
- HIV/AIDS
- inflammation
- insomnia
- kidney disease
- lupus
- migraines
- multiple sclerosis
- Parkinson's disease
- post-concussion syndrome
- PTSD
- residual limb pain

- seizures, especially those characteristic of epilepsy
- Tourette's syndrome
- awful brain injury
- ulcerative colitis

WHAT FORMS DOES CBD COME IN

Anyone who's heard the recent hype about CBD may wonder what forms of CBD there are. CBD, or cannabidiol, is a compound that comes from the cannabis plant. Though cannabis is marijuana, CBD doesn't contain the THC component that provides a high.

Instead, it's used for a variety of therapeutic purposes such as relief of pain and anxiety.

CBD comes in a variety of forms. Some are more effective than others. Here are some of the most common and useful types of CBD delivery.

Oils and Tinctures

CBD oil is made when cannabidiol is extracted from the cannabis plant and infused with a carrier oil such as coconut oil or hempseed oil. This is also known as a tincture.

Oils and tinctures are liquids infused with herbs to be consumed. The most effective way to take CBD in this form is by placing drops directly under the tongue. It's also possible to put them in food or beverage to be consumed.

Vape

According to Consumer Reports, another successful form of CBD use is through vaping. In vaping, the CBD comes in the form of "vape juice" put in a gadget known as a pen.

The user then inhales the item through the vape pen. Vaping, or inhaling the cannabidiol, works well in delivering CBD quickly to the bloodstream.

Edibles

Those who are sensitive to particular tastes or textures might prefer to take their CBD in the form of edibles. These are just as they sound. Edibles are foods infused with cannabidiol. Edibles are also easy to take on the go. They come in several forms of CBD.

Some of the most popular are gummies, chocolates, caramels and baked products. Edibles are discreet and easy to take throughout the day for those who need to spread out higher dosages of CBD.

Eating CBD edibles does take a bit longer to absorb into the bloodstream than some other methods. Typically, individuals can expect to feel effects approximately a half-hour after ingestion.

Topical

Cannabidiol products can be used topically to relieve torment. Balms, salves, creams and lotions made with CBD oil can relieve pain such as aching muscles and joints.

It may additionally be used to improve skin issues. These topical arrangements are absorbed through the skin's cannabinoid receptors to deliver effective alleviation to the targeted area.

Many consider this to be one of the most natural and effective pain relief options around. It's quite well known with athletes and others who wish to avoid prescription or chemical pain relief.

Those with conditions such as joint pain, fibromyalgia and psoriasis may obtain relief through the use of CBD topical treatments.

These are some of the more normal and respected ways to use CBD. Search for testimonials and research to find the most reputable products. Keep these suggestions in mind when thinking about what forms of CBD are there and choose the ones that best meet your lifestyle needs and preferences

HOW CBD OIL HEALS

CBD oil has become one of the world's most talked about and studied remedies for a host of medical and mental conditions.

Vast amounts of evidence show it to be beneficial in the treatment of pain, inflammation, diseases, and mental disorders of all types. It is safe, legal in most locales, and it works.

Scientists have discovered another transmission framework past neurotransmitters that is similarly important for the proper health and functioning of humans.

It is called the endocannabinoid system, and it plays an integral role in our daily lives, influencing everything from mood, appetite, pain perception, fertility and much more.

Our bodies already have cannabinoids and cannabinoid receptors as part of this system, yet now and again, just as neurotransmitters malfunction, our cannabinoid system malfunctions as well.

It turns out that certain plants have cannabinoids as indeed, called phytocannabinoids, which begin from maryjane and hemp. When phytocannabinoids are introduced into the human body, they go to work in remarkable ways to keep our bodies in a state of optimum health

VARIATIONS IN CBD OILS

Of all the personal products now being manufactured from hemp, CBD oil is by far at the top of the list. This term is interchangeable too, as some CBD oils are showcased to be used topically, and others are marketed to be ingested.

Ingestible come in tinctures, extracts, capsules and are sold as CBD oil or Hemp oil. Additionally, some users benefit from CBD oil by using a vaporizer and inhaling it for faster results and better potency.

Notably, there are also wide variations in the quality and usefulness of different brands. There are many online retailers selling CBD oil, yet a closer look at the active ingredients in many of these items show that they contain somewhat little, if any Cannabidiol.

One way purchasers can get duped into buying an inadequate item is with the lack of steady labeling. A common mistake is that consumers assume that Hemp oil and CBD oil are the same. They are not.

Hemp oil and hempseed oil contain Omega 3's, B vitamins, magnesium and other healthy ingredients much like olive oil or coconut oil. Considered a food ingredient, it is legal everywhere and can be used in plans or taken as a supplement.

While good for you, it has none of the medicinal properties of CBD oil. If you purchase hemp oil from a retailer to treat chronic pain or some other condition, you will be disappointed.

CBD oil derived from hemp is purely medicinal, requires more sophisticated methods of extraction, and is much more expensive to produce.

It is made using either a CO_2 extraction method or an ethanol extraction method. These are the only two ways to separate the cannabinoids from the plant material.

For various reasons, CO_2 extraction is preferable. However, ethanol extraction is sufficient, provided that the solvents used are safe. Being aware of the method of extraction will help you choose the best product.

CBD AND NEUROPATHIC PAIN

While an assessed 20 million Americans battle with fringe neuropathy — a medical condition portrayed by nerve damage to the fringe nervous framework, which is the communication network that exists between the central nervous system (the brain and spinal cord) and the rest of the body—

the National Institute of Neurological Disorders and Stroke (NINDS) indicates that this number is likely much higher as not all are reported and some are even misdiagnosed.

The NINDS goes on to explain that this type of neuropathy has a number of potential causes. Among them are:

- Physical injury or trauma, such as after an auto accident
- Diabetes
- Certain cancers and chemotherapy drugs
- Vascular and blood problems
- Autoimmune diseases and infections
- Hormonal and nutritional imbalances
- Kidney and liver disorders

All of these circumstances can be troublesome on their own, however add fringe neuropathy to the mix and it can dramatically affect quality of life.

NEUROPATHY AND QUALITY OF LIFE

When neuropathy involves damage to the motor nerves, quality of life is diminished in that some patients experience muscle shortcoming, uncontrolled jerking, and painful cramps as indicated by the NINDS.

Damage to the sensory nerves of the fringe apprehensive system, on the other hand, can result in life-altering symptoms such as reduced feeling of touch (which can affect balance), increased torment sensations to stimuli that wouldn't typically cause agony, and trouble controlling pain, further compounding torment the board as a whole.

Lastly, when it is the autonomic nerves that are damaged, symptoms may incorporate excess sweating, blood pressure issues, and gastrointestinal trouble. How do you treat these different neuropathic symptoms?

NEUROPATHY TREATMENT OPTION

The NINDS indicates that the first step is to identify and treat the fundamental cause, thus automatically alleviating some of neuropathy's most troubling side effects. Other options include utilizing mechanical aids such as hand and foot braces, taking prescriptions, engaging in transcutaneous electrical nerve stimulation (TENS), and possibly even surgery.

However, numerous people struggling with neuropathy decide to engage in reciprocal and alternative meds as indicated by the NINDS. This includes needle therapy, massage, cognitive conduct therapy, and herbal medications.

It is in this last category that CBD oil would fall. What is CBD oil and how does it work?

CBD stands for cannabidiol, a compound located in the cannabis plant that has been linked to a variety of health benefits, some of which include pain management and relief, fighting inflammation, reduced drug withdrawals, easing epileptic seizures, fighting cancer, lowering anxiety, protecting against blood sugar issues such as type 1 diabetes, slowing the progression of Alzheimer's disease, and more.

Unlike tetrahydrocannabinol (THC), CBD is a compound within the hemp plant that has non-psychoactive properties, meaning that it won't create the high impact most commonly associated with clinical marijuana.

The way CBD works is by communicating with the body's endocannabinoid system and research reveals that this particular system plays an significant role in directing both health and disease.

Essentially, CBD helps bolster the immune system and create a mitigating response based on its association with the cannabinoid receptors known as

CB1 receptors and CBD2 receptors.

Specifically, when CBD is introduced in the endocannabinoid system, it makes positive responses within the fringe anxious system and central apprehensive system, such as pain relief. This relief is noted with multiple types of pain, some of which include chronic pains such as nerve pain (neuropathic pain) or even cancer pain.

Research has confirmed that CBD items can help diminish pain. Truth be told, one 2018 review distributed in the diary Cannabis and Cannabinoid Research found that the top three medical conditions that caused people to use CBD were torment, tension, and depression.

This study also found that 36 percent of the respondents reported that this specific hemp plant extract works "very well by itself" when it comes to easing their medical conditions, with just 4.3 percent stating that, for them, it worked "not very well."

A recent report adds that many pieces of research have also noted that cannabinoids offer benefits specifically for "difficult to treat torment." For case, specialists reference how Canada approved a weed determined nasal spray called Sativex in 2005 for relieving focal neuropathic pain in people with multiple sclerosis.

An application was likewiSe made to the U.S. Food and Drug Administration (FDA) in 2006 so research could be conducted on Sativex to learn its effects on cancer pain.

These researchers further state that "cannabinoid analgesics have for the most part been well tolerated in clinical preliminaries with acceptable adverse event profiles." In other words, there are very limited side effects associated with CBD use. Among the most common are dry mouth, dizziness, nausea, and exhaustion, yet these side effects are typically not strong enough to cause users to suspend CBD use.

NEUROPATHIC PAIN AND CBD OIL FOR ALL

NATURAL PAIN RELIEF

One of the principal benefits of using CBD products in the treatment of neuropathic pain is that it reduces the reliance on pain medication. This is particularly important since the Centers for Disease Control and Prevention reports that, in the United States alone, around 130 individuals pass on every single day due to opioid overdose.

Over-the-counter torment drugs aren't much better when it comes to overall health. For occurrence, research distributed in the journal Annals of Long-Term Care states that chronic use of nonsteroidal anti-inflammatory drugs (NSAIDs) increase more seasoned adults' chances of peptic ulcer disease, intense renal failure, and stroke or myocardial infarction.

This category of pain killers can additionally further irritate chronic sicknesses and potentially interact with prescription medications like blood thinners and corticosteroids.

Using CBD for neuropathic pain instead evades these types of common and possibly risky issues, making it a effective treatment option.

FULL SPECTRUM CBD OIL VS CBD ISOLATE

When utilizing CBD oil for neuropathic torment the executives, you have two general options: full range CBD and CBD isolate.

The Ministry of Hemp states that full spectrum CBD oil refers to oil that, in option to containing CBD, also contains different mixtures found inside the pot plant, such as other cannabinoids and terpenes, the latter of which refers to the oils within the cannabis plant that give it its unmistakable smell. That's why this type of CBD is frequently referred to as "whole plant" oil as, with full spectrum CBD items, the remove is got from compounds taken from the whole hemp plant.

CBD separate, on the other hand, is the term used to describe items that contain almost 100% or more pure CBD as per the Ministry, with no other dynamic ingredients included. Which is better?

Full spectrum CBD oil items have the advantage says the Ministry, chiefly on the grounds that they have more hemp plant compounds and, therefore, are able to offer users more medical advantages as each compound gives unique, positive interactions with the endocannabinoid system.

Research conducted on the Cannabis sativa strain of the cannabis plant approves this, further making sense of that it is the cooperative energy of all of the compounds together that provide such a positive effect.

HOW TO USE CBD OIL FOR NEUROPATHY

When taking full range CBD oil for neuropathic pain, it's best to take it sublingually, which means applying it under the tongue and letting the body absorb it from there. The reason this strategy works best is related to bioavailability, or how well your body is able to assimilate and utilize the hemp oil.

Bioavailability has been a huge concern with dietary supplements in general, with both older adults and pediatric patients both at greater risk of insufficient eating routine and ailing health. However, just because supplements can be taken to help reduce these risks, this doesn't mean that the body retains all of the ingredients they contain, rendering them incapable at solving the problem.

If a supplement it taken orally, for instance, some of the helpful ingredients can be metabolized during the digestive process, leaving less of them for the body to use.

The same is genuine when using CBD oil for neuropathy. To get the most out of it, creating a more positive impact on your neuropathic pain, it's best to take it under the tongue.

When your goal is pain management, it's likewise useful to combine CBD oil with a quality skin CBD cream. While the CBD oil interacts with CBD receptors body-wide, the topical cream empowers you to better direct your therapy to the area or areas that hurt the most.

CBD DOSAGE

Another factor to consider when taking CBD oil for neuropathic pain is that, commonly, people don't take a high enough dose of CBD and, subsequently, mistakenly think it doesn't work for them.

HOW MUCH SHOULD YOU TAKE?

Researchers from the Research Institute of the McGill University Health Center and McGill University in Quebec, Canada, state that, after conducting different investigations on animals, "low portions of CBD administered for seven days alleviate both pain and tension, two symptoms often associated in neuropathic or ongoing pain."

Starting with these lower doses empowers you to see what sway the CBD oil is having on your neuropathic torment without taking more than you need. You can always scale up from there if you're not seeing the results you desire, increasing your dosage until your torment begins to subside.

CBD TO POTENTIALLY

RELIEVE STROKES

The mitigating and neuroprotective properties of CBD enable it to prevent auto-immune attacks on the brain tissues and to prevent the passing of brain cells. Being an antioxidant, CBD helps in removing toxins and dead blood cells from blood vessels.
It also lowers bad cholesterol levels while increasing good cholesterol. All of these properties are essential for improving mind health.

Additionally, separated from helping with pain management after stroke or TBI, CBD helps in protecting neurons and body tissue.

Currently, there are various CBD products that can be purchased online. They include CBD crystals, CBD edibles, CBD oil, and CBD wax among others. Take time to learn about these products on this website before you decide on the item that is right for you.

HOW CBD SHIELD THE BRAIN AFTER EXPERIENCING THIS DISEASE

When you experience a stroke, your body undergoes an intense process of inflammation where the hemorrhage or clot happened. Here comes the role of cannabidiol.

CBD (Cannabidiol) can guard your mind by inhibiting certain mechanisms.

It can lower the level of cytokine as well as stops the inflammatory immune response, which can kill the active brain cells.

Along with mitigating effects, it may also have potent antioxidant effects.

With its antioxidant properties, it counteracts the unnecessary cellular oxidation.

Moreover, it also takes away the dead cells, as well as toxins from the blood vessels.

IS CBD OIL USEFUL TO RECOVER FROM THIS DISEASE

CBD oil can help treat this ailment. Lowering and balancing the cholesterol level is necessary because if its level increases, then the possibility of having this disease also increases.

CBD can lower the unwanted cholesterol level and balance the cholesterol level. Thus, the risk of having an embolic stroke decreases.

Moreover, cannabidiol can recuperate the motor abilities as it can increase the blood flow to the damaged areas.

Cannabidiol hemp oil can be a powerful option to recover from this disease in light of the fact that it binds actively with the receptors across the ECS. It may also consist of useful qualities in enhancing cerebral blood flow.

In addition to this, the component also plays a vital job in hindering the oxidation, irritation, as well as, in promoting overall function and health within the endocannabinoid system.

CBD OIL AND STROKE

PAIN

During a stroke, uneasiness and pain occur on the patient's body (one side of the body). Moreover, in this stage, large parts of the nervous system and brain lack oxygen.

This, in turn, causes a wide-scale as well as massive death of cells, including the cells that enable your body to sense and process pain.

When there is damage to the cells, there will be serious neurological damage, which causes neuropathic pain.

Using CBD oil for stroke victims can be a natural, effective, and safe solution to oversee its symptoms. It's because this compound binds with the CB1 receptor present in the endocannabinoid system. This receptor can manage a sense of pain.

As CBD ties with this receptor, it affects directly to the source of pain in an effective way and can help the sufferer to carry on with a quality life

FOODS THAT CAN HELP PEOPLE RECOVER FROM STROKE

Blueberries: These berries are popular because of their memory-improvement qualities. As per the studies, blueberries have the efficiency to improve cognitive functions due to the effects of flavanoids on the cell signaling paths.

Tomatoes: Tomatoes contain antioxidant lycopene, which offers neuroprotective benefits as well as lessen the sway of brain damage occurring in rats due to ischemic stroke.

Beans: This is a source of glucose to the brain. In addition to this, they also help to stabilize the level of your blood glucose. This, in turn, balances the glucose supply to brain.

Pomegranate: Consuming pomegranates will help you to safeguard yourself from the damage occurring due to free radicals, as they are antioxidants. Thus, pomegranates can be useful for stroke recovery.

Seeds and Nuts: These are a perfect source of vitamin E, an antioxidant.

Eating flaxseeds or walnuts is good as they both are a wellspring of omega-3s (brain boosters).

HEALING OPTIONS FOR THIS AILMENT

To recuperate from this disease, proper and immediate medical care is necessary.

Treatment for this depends on its type.

Let's have a more in-depth look into it.

TRADITIONAL MEDICINES FOR THIS AILMENT

Here are the conventional medicines for treating this disease:

Antiplatelet Medicines: These medicines prevent blood clots by not allowing the blood platelets to bond together. Clopidogrel and aspirin are the most common antiplatelet medicines.

Tissue Plasminogen Activator: This is emergency medicine, which comes into use during a stroke to prevent the blood clot causing this health problem.

Satins: This is the most common medication prescribed by doctors in the United States. Satins put an end to the production of the enzyme, which can turn the cholesterol into plaque, a stick, and thick substance, which can develop on the walls of arteries and can cause strokes as well as heart attacks.

Anticoagulants: These medicines have the effectiveness to reduce the ability of blood from clotting. Warfarin is a popular anticoagulant.

Blood Pressure Medicines: Controlling the high level of pulse can help to prevent this disease. This is because high blood pressure can lead to the development of plaque in your arteries, which can result in a stroke.

NUTRIENTS AND VITAMINS TO REDUCE THE RISK OF THIS DISEASE

Betaine: According to investigate, amino acid betaine can reduce homocysteine levels.

Vitamin B-6, Vitamin B-12, and Folic Acid: Some B vitamin supplements can lower the levels of amino acid homocysteine. Lowering the amino acid homocysteine level is necessary as it can increase the possibility of this disease.

Vitamin E: Consuming vitamin E supplements can help to manage the memory impairment.

Vitamin C: Taking vitamin C supplements can help repair the damage in the blood vessel as well as reduce the development of plaque in the arteries.

Vitamin D: Vitamin D supplements can play a significant role in lessening the risk of this disease. It's because having a low level of vitamin D can increase the possibility of artery-blocking strokes, mainly in folks with a high level of blood pressure.

Magnesium: Mineral magnesium can lower the level of blood pressure.

Omega-3 Fatty Acids: These fatty acids can improve the level of cholesterol.

ALTERNATIVE THERAPIES FOR THIS DISORDER

Tai Chi: This is a ancient Chinese traditional therapy, which incorporates a series of stretches as well as slow developments along with deep breathing. As per the researches, this therapy can help the stroke sufferers in improving balance.

Aromatherapy: Studies show that this method can be a worthy alternative for the patients suffering this ailment.

Yoga: Yoga can help to improve coordination as well as balance-the two common problems that the stroke patients experience after a stroke.

Massage Therapy: According to a study published in the Journal of Chinese Integrative Medicine, herbal treatments, as well as Thai massage, can perk up the rest patterns, everyday work, chronic pain, and mood in stroke victims.

Acupuncture: This is a ancient Chinese complementary medication, which is a potent alternative way to recover from this disease.

HERBAL ALTERNATIVES FOR TREATING THIS

DISORDER

Turmeric: This can reduce the level of cholesterol and help to avoid the blockages in arteries.

Garlic: Garlic can prevent blood clotting as well as destroy plaque.

Ashwagandha: Ashwagandha can prevent as well as cure stroke as it has antioxidant properties.

Gotu Kola: This is a herb, which can boost the mental function in folks suffering from this illness.

Bilberry: This can lessen the level of blood sugar and improve cholesterol.

When discussing herbal alternatives, we want to mention Cannabidiol (CBD) as well. Making Use of CBD oil for stroke recovery as well as prevention can be a promising option.

SIDE EFFECTS AND SAFETY CONCERN OF CBD

CBD has a good safety profile. It isn't addictive, and you can't overdose on CBD. However, there are still a few important things to keep in mind if you want to try CBD.

Possible side effects

- fatigue
- diarrhea
- changes in appetite

- changes in weight

CBD could interact with other drugs. That's because CBD may interfere with certain liver enzymes. This interference could stop the liver from metabolizing other drugs or substances, leading to higher concentrations of them in your system.

That's why it's important to talk to your doctor about any potential drug interactions before taking CBD.

CBD could increase your risk of liver toxicity. A recent study has raised concerns about CBD's potential for liver damage. Researchers suggest that CBD affects the liver in a similar way as alcohol, some medications, and even certain dietary supplements.

CBD NOT WORKING FOR YOU

Your CBD product isn't from a reputable source

WHERE DID YOU BUY YOUR CBD OIL?

As it grows in popularity, it seems like CBD is popping up all over — from online companies to over-the-counter shops. You might have even tried a free sample to see if it works without investing anything more than the cost of shipping.

Unfortunately, some of these products don't have high-quality CBD. The Food and Drug Administration (FDA) hasn't yet approved any nonprescription CBD products.

Some scammers take full advantage of that fact by selling low-quality products that aren't labeled accurately.

One group of specialists analyzed 84 CBD products and found that only 31 percent of them contained the sum of CBD that had been advertised.

So the next time you're looking to invest in a new CBD product, use these three tips to make sure the product lives up to its promises:

Many CBD users have reported trying several different brands before settling on one that works for them, so keep searching if your first try doesn't produce the results you're looking for.

You need to fabricate it up in your system

Finding the right dosage of CBD can be a tricky endeavor. The appropriate amount varies for each individual, as every person has an unique science that results in a different reaction.

SO HOW DO YOU FIGURE OUT WHAT'S RIGHT FOR YOU?

Start with an low dose and gradually increase it over time until you find your sweet spot.

Some folks find that taking a daily portion can help sustain a level of CBD in your body, which might stimulate your endocannabinoid system (more on what this is, underneath) to make it react more to cannabinoids like CBD.

And many people use a micro dosing technique to find their personal dosage and adjust it as required over time.

You may find it helpful to use a journal to log your results.

Keep track of how much you've taken, how you feel before dosing and at several time intervals afterward, and any changes in symptoms that you notice.

Over time, this data can help paint a picture of how CBD affects you.

You need to give it more time

The first time I tried CBD, I wondered if I'd wasted my money on some overhyped trend. I put some drops of an oil tincture under my tongue, expected near-instant relief from my chronic pain, and got... nothing.

My experience isn't at all unusual, because immediate results aren't all that common.

In fact, many people take CBD for a few weeks or even several months before they see a difference.

Exploring the effects of CBD isn't as simple as taking a couple of Tylenol and calling it a day. It actually requires a certain level of commitment to put time and thought into your process of uncovering the long-term effects.

If you're still not seeing results after a while (think a few months), then it might be time to move on and try a different brand. Your CBD journal can help you keep track of how long it's been and whether or not you've experienced any changes.

Patience is key, and while it can be frustrating to keep attempting with no results, you may end up feeling super grateful that you didn't give up.

You need a different delivery system

It seems like I'm hearing about a new CBD product just about every week. You can find everything from CBD coffee to shower salts and lube.

So if you've been trying one delivery system with no luck, it's possible that an alternate form would work better for you.

One factor to consider is bioavailability, which essentially refers to how much of the CBD actually gets into your bloodstream.

For model, if you eat CBD gummies, they have to go through your stomach related tract before you can absorb them, and the amount that winds up in your system may be generally low.

On the other hand, if you take a tincture sublingually — which means under the tongue — you're absorbing it directly into your bloodstream. So you could get quicker, more noticeable results than you would from waiting for your digestive system to process it.

IT'S JUST NOT FOR YOU

CBD may be popular, however that doesn't mean it's a miracle drug that will work for everyone. After all of your efforts, it's possible that you'll find that CBD simply doesn't work for you.

Your level of absorption and reaction to CBD depends on a variety of factors including your:

- metabolism
- biochemistry
- genetics

Your endocannabinoid system is the framework in your body that associates with the active compounds in cannabis, and each person's works a little differently.

If you have that mutation, you might be prone to lower levels of anxiety, however because you already have extra endocannabinoids you could not see much of a difference when you take CBD.

And if you have persistent friends, don't be afraid to tell them to stop bugging you about giving CBD an attempt. After all, there's no such thing as a one-size-fits-all treatment!

CONCLUSION

Chronic pain conditions are often baffling conditions for patients and doctors alike. Neuropathic torment is a complex condition that arises from problems with nerve flagging and can be caused by harm to the peripheral or central nervous system.

Symptoms of this type of pain can vary and this condition is often challenging for doctors to diagnosis.

Various treatment options exist for the treatment of neuropathic pain; however, treatment frequently only provides some relief for many patients.

Patients are energized to speak with their physician to determine what treatment will provide them with the most effective torment relief from this crippling condition.

Made in the USA
Las Vegas, NV
02 March 2024